Women's Guide to Multi-Orgasmic Sex

A Comprehensive Guide for Women to Achieving Multi-Orgasmic Sex, Mastering Pleasure, and Embracing Sexual Empowerment for Lifelong Fulfillment and Intimate Connection

Cheryl Bach

Women's Guide to Multi-Orgasmic Sex

Publisher: IntimateInk Press

Email: intimateinkpress@gmail.com

This book is a work of nonfiction intended for informational purposes only. The content of this book is based on the author's research, knowledge, and experience, and it is provided with the understanding that the author and publisher are not engaged in rendering legal, medical, or professional advice. The information in this book is not a substitute for professional guidance or assistance. Readers should consult with relevant professionals for advice and assistance regarding their specific situations. The author and publisher disclaim any liability for any loss or risk, personal or otherwise, which is incurred as a consequence, directly or indirectly, of the use and application of any of the contents of this book.

Cover design by IntimateInk Press

Interior layout and design by IntimateInk Press

Printed in USA

Fonts: Google fonts

Image: Freepik.com. This cover has been designed using assets from Freepik.com

For permission to use copyrighted material from this book, please contact the copyright holder listed above.

First Edition: 2024

Distributed by Amazon.com, Inc.

Cheryl Bach

Table of Contents

Women's Guide to Multi-Orgasmic Sex

Chapter I.

Introduction

This comprehensive guide is designed for women who want to explore their sexuality and take charge of their own sexual wellbeing. Whether you're single or in a relationship, this book will provide you with the tools and techniques you need to achieve multi-orgasmic sex, master pleasure, and embrace sexual empowerment for lifelong fulfillment and intimate connection.

Multi-Orgasmic Sex and Why it Is Important for Women

Multi-orgasmic sex is a term used to describe the ability to achieve multiple orgasms during one sexual encounter. Unlike men who typically experience a refractory period after orgasm, women are capable of experiencing multiple orgasms without needing a break in between. While some women naturally possess this ability, others may need to learn and practice specific techniques to achieve it. This book will guide you through the process of becoming multi-orgasmic and help you harness the power of your sexuality to achieve deeper levels of pleasure and connection.

Cultural Stigma Surrounding Female Sexuality

Unfortunately, female sexuality has long been stigmatized by our culture. Women are often portrayed as either prudish or promiscuous, with little room for exploration and experimentation. This stigma has created a barrier that prevents women from fully embracing their sexuality and experiencing the full spectrum of pleasure and intimacy that is possible.

That's why it's important to take a proactive approach to your own sexual exploration and become empowered in your own sexuality. By embracing your desires, exploring your body, and discussing your needs with partners, you can break through societal stigmas and achieve a more fulfilling, satisfying, and empowered sex life.

Importance of Self-Discovery, Pleasure, and Empowerment for Women

At the heart of this guide is the belief that women deserve to experience the full spectrum of pleasure and connection that is possible through sex. Pleasure is not something to be ashamed of or hidden away but is instead a natural and necessary part of our physical and emotional wellbeing. Through self-discovery, mindfulness and relaxation techniques, communication with partners, and specific techniques for achieving multiple orgasms, you can achieve a deeper level of pleasure that will enhance your overall quality of life.

This guide will provide you with a comprehensive toolkit for achieving multi-orgasmic sex. You'll learn the anatomy and physiology of female sexuality, including the clitoris and other erogenous zones, and how to explore and stimulate these areas to increase your own pleasure. You'll also gain a deeper understanding of the complexities of sexual desire and arousal, and how to control these sensations to prevent overstimulation or discomfort.

We'll delve into the importance of communication with partners, and provide strategies for effective communication that ensure both partners' needs are met. We'll discuss mutual pleasure techniques, including techniques and toys that can be incorporated into sexual experiences to enhance pleasure for both partners. This includes strategies for achieving multiple orgasms, both alone and with partners.

Throughout this guide, we'll emphasize the importance of sexual empowerment and liberation, which involves embracing female sexuality and rejecting shame or stigma. By gaining a deeper understanding of your own body and desires, you can become more confident in your sexuality and express your needs and boundaries more effectively.

Finally, we'll discuss the importance of sexual health and safety, including strategies for maintaining sexual health, such as regular STI testing and contraceptive use. We'll also emphasize the importance of seeking medical help for any concerns or issues related to sexual health.

In short, this guide is designed to provide you with comprehensive information and useful tips for achieving multi-orgasmic sex, mastering pleasure, and embracing sexual empowerment and fulfillment. Through self-discovery and effective communication with partners, you can take charge of your own sexual wellbeing and achieve deep levels of pleasure and connection. By breaking through cultural stigmas and celebrating your own sexuality, you can achieve a greater sense of fulfillment and satisfaction in your life.

We hope this guide serves as a valuable resource and empowers you to take your sex life to the next level.

Chapter II.

Self-Discovery

One of the keys to achieving multi-orgasmic sex is a deeper understanding of your own body and desires. Through self-discovery, you can explore what brings you pleasure and discover new ways to enhance sexual experiences. In this chapter, we will discuss the importance of self-discovery in achieving multi-orgasmic sex. Understanding your own body, sexual preferences, and desires is a crucial step towards unlocking the full potential of your sexual experiences.

Exploring Personal Desires and Preferences

To begin exploring your personal desires and preferences, try setting aside some quiet time for yourself to reflect on your own sexual experiences. Consider what you enjoy most about them, what feels pleasurable, and what leaves you feeling unsatisfied.

It may also be helpful to experiment with different techniques, positions, and forms of stimulation either on your own or with a partner. This experimentation can help you discover new forms of pleasure and learn what you enjoy most.

Discussion of the Clitoris and Other Erogenous Zones

Understanding your body's anatomy is an integral part of self-discovery. The clitoris is one of the most critical erogenous zones that play a significant role in female sexual pleasure. It's highly sensitive to touch and stimulation and can lead to intense orgasms.

Cheryl Bach

When exploring your clitoris, try experimenting with different types of stimulation, such as light touches, circular motions, or direct pressure. Pay attention to what feels pleasurable and what doesn't. It's also important to communicate with your partner about what type of touch and pressure feels good to you.

There are other erogenous zones present in the female body, such as the inner thighs, nipples, and neck, which can be explored during sex and are known to increase pleasure. Learning how to stimulate these areas and exploring which ones feel the most pleasurable for you is a crucial part of self-discovery. You can explore these areas on your own or with a partner to understand what feels good to you.

Educating Yourself about Anatomy and Masturbation Techniques

Educating yourself about your body's anatomy, including its physical and physiological aspects, is an essential part of self-discovery. When you understand the structure and function of your reproductive system, you will have a better understanding of how it functions sexually.

Masturbation is a great way to explore your body and learn more about yourself sexually. It's also a way to practice self-love and develop a deeper sense of intimacy with yourself. Try experimenting with different techniques such as using a vibrator or stimulating different parts of your body.

As you explore new masturbation techniques, pay close attention to what feels pleasurable. It's essential to be patient and gentle with yourself, taking your time to explore different sensations and enjoying the moment. You can also use this time to identify when you're most aroused, what types of stimulation you enjoy, and what kind of fantasies or thoughts help you achieve arousal.

It's important to keep in mind that everyone's preferences and desires are unique, and exploring what works for you can be both exciting and liberating. Take the time to learn about your body and what brings you pleasure, and don't be afraid to communicate your needs and boundaries with your partner to enhance your sexual experiences together.

In conclusion, self-discovery is a critical step towards achieving multi-orgasmic sex and mastering pleasure. By exploring personal desires and preferences, discussing the clitoris and other erogenous zones, and educating yourself about anatomy and masturbation techniques, you can develop a deeper sense of intimacy with yourself and your partner. This exploration can help you unlock the full potential of your sexual experiences, enhance pleasure, and build a strong foundation for long-lasting fulfillment and intimate connection.

Remember, there's no right or wrong way to explore your body or your desires. It's natural to have questions or uncertainties, and taking the time to explore your sexuality can be an exciting and liberating journey. Be open to new experiences, communicate your needs, and always prioritize your own pleasure and satisfaction.

In the following chapters, we will discuss techniques and strategies for achieving multi-orgasmic sex, including breathing exercises, pelvic floor exercises, and exploring sexual fantasies. By building on the foundation of self-discovery discussed in this chapter, you'll be well on your way to achieving a deep sense of intimacy, connection, and fulfillment through multi-orgasmic sex.

Chapter III.

Mindfulness and Relaxation Techniques

In this chapter, we will discuss the importance of mindfulness and relaxation techniques in achieving multi-orgasmic sex. By learning how to quiet the mind and reduce anxiety and distractions, you can enhance pleasure, build intimacy with your partner, and achieve deeper levels of sexual fulfillment.

Breathing Exercises

Breathing exercises are powerful tools for calming the body and reducing stress and anxiety levels. By focusing on your breath, you can decrease heart rate, lower blood pressure, and promote a sense of calm and relaxation.

To begin, find a comfortable seated position and close your eyes. Take several deep, slow breaths in through your nose and out through your mouth, exhaling fully each time. Visualize inhaling positive energy and exhaling negative energy with each breath.

As you continue to breathe, try to focus on the sensation of air moving in and out of your body. Feel your chest and abdomen expand with each inhale and deflate with each exhale. If your mind starts to wander, bring your attention back to your breath. You can do this exercise for a few minutes each day to help reduce stress and anxiety.

During sex, breathing exercises can also help you stay present in the moment and enhance pleasure. Deep breathing can increase blood flow and sensitivity to erogenous zones, making it easier to achieve orgasm.

Mindfulness Practices

Mindfulness is the act of being present in the moment and fully engaging in the experience at hand, without judgment or distraction. Practicing mindfulness during sex can help you focus on the sensations you're experiencing, build intimacy with your partner, and achieve greater pleasure and fulfillment.

To practice mindfulness during sex, try to focus all of your attention on the physical sensations you're experiencing. Pay attention to the way your body feels, the touch of your partner's skin, and the sounds in the room. Try to let go of any outside distractions or thoughts and be fully present in the moment.

Remember that mindfulness is not about achieving a specific goal or outcome. It's more about being open and attentive to whatever arises during the present moment. With practice, you can learn to apply this same kind of awareness and presence to other areas of your life, beyond sex.

Techniques for Reducing Anxiety and Distractions

Anxiety and external distractions can prevent you from fully experiencing pleasure during sex. Fortunately, there are techniques you can use to help reduce feelings of anxiety and become more focused and present in the moment.

One such technique is progressive muscle relaxation. This involves tensing and relaxing each muscle group in turn, starting at your feet and working your way up to your head. As you tense each muscle group, hold it for a few seconds, then release and allow the muscle to relax fully.

Another technique is visualization. This involves imagining yourself in a peaceful and calming environment, such as a beach or forest, and focusing on the sights, sounds, and sensations around you. By visualizing a peaceful environment, you can help reduce feelings of anxiety and distraction.

It's also important to communicate with your partner and establish clear boundaries and expectations. Let your partner know if you're feeling anxious or distracted and work together to find ways to overcome these feelings. By creating a safe and supportive environment, you can feel more relaxed and open to experiencing pleasure during sex.

In conclusion, mindfulness and relaxation techniques are powerful tools for achieving multi-orgasmic sex. By taking the time to quiet the mind, reduce anxiety and distractions, and be fully present in the moment, you can enhance pleasure, build intimacy with your partner, and achieve deeper levels of sexual fulfillment.

Remember that these techniques are not quick fixes or one-time solutions. They require practice and patience to master. Incorporating mindfulness and relaxation practices into your daily routine can help you stay calm and focused, reduce stress and anxiety levels, and enhance your overall wellbeing.

In the next chapter, we will discuss the role of communication and consent in achieving multi-orgasmic sex. By fostering open communication, setting clear boundaries, and respecting each other's needs and desires, you can build a strong foundation for intimacy and connection with your partner.

Chapter IV.

Communication and Mutual Pleasure

In this chapter, we will discuss the importance of open communication with partners about desires and boundaries in achieving multi-orgasmic sex. By communicating your needs and desires effectively, you can build a strong foundation for intimacy and connection, as well as enhance pleasure for both yourself and your partner.

Importance of Open Communication

Open communication is essential for creating a safe and supportive environment for sexual exploration. By letting your partner know what you like and don't like, you can build trust and intimacy, and avoid misunderstandings or discomfort. It's important to have conversations about sexual health, boundaries, and expectations before engaging in sexual activity, and to continue these conversations throughout your relationship.

By being honest and transparent with your partner, you can also build a deeper sense of sexual empowerment and confidence. Knowing that your partner respects your needs and desires can help you feel more comfortable and confident in expressing them.

One important aspect of open communication is consent. It's essential to always ask for and respect your partner's consent before engaging in any sexual activity, and to check in with them throughout the experience to ensure that both parties are comfortable and consenting. Remember that consent must be enthusiastic and ongoing, and that it can be withdrawn at any time.

Strategies for Effective Communication

Effective communication involves more than just talking. It also includes non-verbal cues and active listening. When you're communicating with your partner about your desires and boundaries, consider using the following strategies:

Non-Verbal Cues: Pay attention to your body language and facial expressions, as they can communicate a lot about your feelings and desires. Make eye contact, touch your partner affectionately, and use gentle gestures to indicate your interest and attraction. You can also guide your partner's touches and movements with your hands or body, and moan or breathe heavily to indicate what feels good.

Active Listening: Effective communication also involves active listening, which means paying close attention to what your partner is saying and responding thoughtfully. Paraphrase your partner's words to ensure that you understand them correctly, and ask clarifying questions if necessary. Avoid interrupting or dismissing your partner's feelings, and make an effort to respond in a supportive and empathetic way.

Mutual Pleasure

Multi-orgasmic sex is not just about achieving pleasure for one person; it's about enhancing pleasure for both partners. By focusing on mutual pleasure, you can create a more satisfying and fulfilling sexual experience for both yourself and your partner.

Some techniques that can enhance mutual pleasure include:

Exploration: Take the time to explore each other's bodies and find out what feels good. Touch, kiss, and caress your partner in different ways to discover their sensitive spots and preferred touch.

Communication: Ask your partner what they like and what they want. Encourage them to communicate their desires and needs, and be open and responsive to their requests.

Variety: Change things up regularly to keep things exciting. Try different positions, techniques, and settings to keep the experience fresh and enjoyable.

Foreplay: Don't rush into things. Spend plenty of time on foreplay activities, such as kissing, touching, and oral sex, to build arousal and enhance pleasure for both partners.

Focus on mutual pleasure: During sex, focus on pleasuring each other rather than just yourself. Take turns focusing on each other and experiment with different techniques that feel good for both partners. By prioritizing mutual pleasure, you can strengthen your connection and intimacy, and reach higher levels of sexual fulfillment.

It's also important to remember that pleasure is not just physical, but emotional and psychological as well. By being present and fully engaged in the experience, you can deepen your connection with your partner and foster a sense of emotional intimacy, which can enhance pleasure and satisfaction.

In conclusion, effective communication and mutual pleasure are essential components of multi-orgasmic sex. By being open and honest with your partner about your desires and boundaries, and focusing on enhancing pleasure for both parties, you can build a strong foundation for intimacy and connection, and achieve deeper levels of sexual fulfillment and empowerment.

Chapter V.

Techniques for Multi-Orgasmic Sex

In this chapter, we will discuss techniques for achieving multi-orgasmic sex. By learning different techniques and approaches to sexual pleasure, you can experience deeper levels of fulfillment and empowerment.

Types of Orgasms

Before discussing techniques for multiple orgasms, let's first explore the different types of orgasms that a woman can experience:

Clitoral orgasm: This is the most common type of orgasm, achieved through direct stimulation of the clitoris.

Vaginal orgasm: This type of orgasm is achieved through stimulation of the G-spot and other sensitive areas inside the vagina.

Combination orgasm: This type of orgasm is achieved through simultaneous stimulation of the clitoris and vagina.

Anal orgasm: This type of orgasm is achieved through stimulation of the anus and rectum. It can be achieved through penetration or anal stimulation with fingers or toys.

Cervical orgasm: This type of orgasm is achieved through deep penetration and stimulation of the cervix.

Nipple orgasm: This type of orgasm is achieved through stimulation of the nipples. Some women can experience nipple orgasms without any genital stimulation.

Cheryl Bach

It's important for women to understand the different types of orgasms in order to explore their own bodies and discover what feels good for them.

Techniques for Achieving Multiple Orgasms

Now, let's discuss techniques for achieving multiple orgasms. Multi-orgasmic sex involves experiencing more than one orgasm during a sexual encounter. With the right techniques and mindset, almost any woman can achieve multiple orgasms.

Here are some techniques to explore:

Build arousal slowly: Don't rush into sex. Take your time to build arousal slowly through foreplay activities, such as kissing, touching, and oral sex. This can help you to achieve a higher level of arousal before moving onto penetration.

Finding the right position: Experiment with different positions to find what feels good for you. Some positions are more likely to stimulate the clitoris or G-spot, which can lead to multiple orgasms. For example, female-on-top and rear-entry positions are often recommended for achieving multiple orgasms.

Relax and let go: For many women, it's important to relax and let go of any mental distractions or anxieties in order to achieve multiple orgasms. Focus on the pleasure that you're feeling and let your body respond spontaneously to sensations.

Try edging: Edging involves bringing yourself close to orgasm and then backing off, allowing your arousal to build slowly over time. This can help you to achieve more intense orgasms and potentially multiple orgasms. Try bringing yourself close to orgasm through clitoral stimulation and then backing off before continuing again.

Cheryl Bach

Take a break: After achieving your first orgasm, take a break before continuing with other activities. This can help you to maintain your arousal and potentially achieve another orgasm later in the session.

Use different techniques for different types of orgasms: Remember that different types of orgasms may require different types of stimulation. Experiment with different techniques to find what works best for you. For example, clitoral stimulation may work best for achieving clitoral orgasms, while G-spot stimulation may be needed for vaginal orgasms.

Controlling Arousal and Avoiding Overstimulation

It's important to control your arousal in order to avoid overstimulation, which can make it more difficult to achieve multiple orgasms.

Here are some tips for controlling and managing arousal:

Focus on your breath: Slow, deep breathing can help you stay relaxed and in control of your arousal levels. Try focusing on your breath during sexual activities to maintain a steady level of arousal.

Take breaks: As mentioned earlier, taking breaks can help you to maintain your arousal rather than becoming overstimulated. Take a few minutes to cuddle, talk, or engage in non-sexual activities before returning to sexual activities.

Slow down: Sometimes slowing down the pace of sexual activities can help you to stay in control of your arousal levels. Taking your time and savoring each moment can help you to achieve multiple orgasms more easily.

Incorporate non-genital areas: Explore other parts of your body that can be pleasurable, such as your neck, ears, and breasts. By incorporating non-genital areas, you can help to spread out your pleasure and avoid becoming overstimulated in one area.

Use different techniques: Using a variety of different sexual techniques and activities can help to keep you interested and engaged, and can help you to achieve multiple orgasms. Experiment with different positions, toys, and foreplay activities to find what works best for you.

Tips for Incorporating Toys and Other Aids

Incorporating sex toys and other aids can be a great way to enhance your sexual experiences and make it easier to achieve multiple orgasms.

Here are some tips for incorporating toys and aids:

Choose the right toy: There are many different types of sex toys available, so it's important to choose the right one for your needs. Consider the type of stimulation you enjoy most and choose a toy that can provide that type of stimulation.

Communicate with your partner: If you're using toys or other aids during sex, it's important to communicate with your partner about what you enjoy and what you want to try. This can help to enhance your experience and make it more enjoyable for both partners.

Use plenty of lubrication: Using plenty of lubrication can help you to avoid discomfort or pain during sex and can make it easier to achieve multiple orgasms. Choose a high-quality lubricant that is safe for use with your toy or aid.

Relax and enjoy: Remember that sex should be enjoyable and pleasurable. Try to relax and enjoy the experience, rather than worrying about achieving multiple orgasms or performing in a certain way.

Cheryl Bach

Chapter VI.

Sexual Empowerment and Liberation

Importance of Embracing Female Sexuality

As women, we have been conditioned to feel shame and stigma surrounding our sexuality. It's essential to recognize and reject these negative messages and embrace the power and joy of our sexuality.

Embracing our sexuality can provide numerous benefits, including:

- Improved self-esteem and body image
- Greater sexual pleasure and fulfillment
- Increased emotional and physical intimacy with partners
- Enhanced sense of self-awareness and personal growth

By embracing our sexuality, we can also challenge harmful societal norms and support a more positive and inclusive sexual culture.

Strategies for Self-Empowerment

Embracing female sexuality can be a journey that requires self-empowerment and self-love.

Here are some strategies for achieving self-empowerment:

Practice Self-Love: We must learn to love and accept ourselves fully, including our bodies, desires, and fantasies. This can involve positive affirmations, self-care practices, and embracing self-expression in all aspects of our lives.

Develop Body Positivity: Society's beauty standards can negatively impact how we view ourselves and our bodies. It's important to reject these standards and embrace body positivity, which means accepting and loving our bodies for what they are, regardless of shape, size, or appearance.

Foster Sexual Exploration: By exploring and discovering our sexual desires and fantasies, we can gain a greater sense of self-awareness, confidence, and empowerment. This can involve solo sex practices, communication with partners, and trying new things in the bedroom.

Discussion of Consent, Boundaries, and Sexual Agency

A crucial aspect of embracing female sexuality is understanding and exercising our sexual agency. This means taking ownership of our bodies and making intentional choices about our sexual experiences.

Consent and boundaries are essential components of sexual agency. We must communicate our boundaries clearly and respect those of our partners. We should never feel pressured or obligated to engage in any sexual activity that we are not comfortable with. Consensual and respectful sexual encounters can lead to increased pleasure, intimacy, and overall satisfaction.

Part of exercising sexual agency includes advocating for ourselves and supporting the autonomy and agency of others. We must reject harmful stereotypes and narratives that perpetuate shame and stigma around female sexuality. Instead, we should embrace and celebrate the sexuality of all individuals, regardless of gender identity or sexual orientation.

Embracing female sexuality requires a commitment to self-reflection, education, and empowerment. By practicing self-love, challenging societal norms, and embracing sexual exploration, we can empower ourselves and take control of our sexual experiences. By prioritizing consent, boundaries, and agency, we can ensure that our sexual encounters are safe, respectful, and fulfilling.

In conclusion, embracing female sexuality is a crucial component of our overall well-being and sense of fulfillment. By rejecting shame and stigma and prioritizing self-love and exploration, we can empower ourselves and take ownership of our sexual experiences. By advocating for ourselves and supporting the autonomy of others, we can create a more positive and inclusive sexual culture. Remember to prioritize your own desires, communicate your boundaries, and celebrate all aspects of your sexuality as you strive towards a lifetime of sexual fulfillment and intimate connection.

Cheryl Bach

Chapter VII.

Sexual Health and Safety

Strategies for Maintaining Sexual Health

As women, it's important that we regularly prioritize our sexual health.

These practices include:

Regular STI testing: It's important to get tested for STIs regularly, whether you have more than one partner or not. Even if symptoms do not present, some STIs can still be present. Make sure to get tested on a routine basis, at least once a year if you are sexually active, and to encourage your partners to do the same.

Contraceptive Use: Using contraceptives such as condoms and other barrier methods can reduce the risk of pregnancy and prevent the transmission of STIs during penetrative sex. Additionally, other forms of contraception, such as hormonal birth control, can prevent pregnancy and regulate menstrual cycles.

Safe Sex Practices

Safe sex practices are crucial in maintaining our sexual health and preventing the transmission of STIs.

These practices include:

Using Condoms or Dental Dams: Male and female condoms are effective barriers that can prevent the spread of STIs during penetrative sex. Dental dams can also be used during oral sex to prevent the transmission of STIs.

Regular Hygiene: Maintaining good hygiene is important for reducing the risk of infections. Make sure to wash your genitals regularly and thoroughly with mild soap and warm water. It's also essential to urinate after sex to flush out any bacteria that may have entered the urethra.

Communication: Clear communication with your partner(s) is important for practicing safe sex. Discussing mutual expectations and boundaries before engaging in sexual activity can help prevent any misunderstandings or unintended consequences. Additionally, you can discuss and agree on what safe sex practices you plan to use.

Seeking Medical Help

If you have any concerns or issues related to your sexual health, it's crucial to seek medical help from a trusted healthcare provider. Issues relating to sexual health can range from minor discomfort to severe infections that require medical attention.

Cheryl Bach

Here are some common issues related to sexual health that you may encounter:

- Vaginal itching or discharge
- Pain or discomfort during sex
- Abnormal bleeding or pain during menstruation
- Pelvic pain or discomfort

It's important not to ignore any of these symptoms and get help as soon as possible to avoid further complications.

Empowering Women

Empowering women to take control of their own sexual health is essential for their overall well-being and sense of fulfillment.

This includes:

Advocating for Yourself: Don't be afraid to speak up when it comes to your sexual health and well-being. If your healthcare provider isn't taking your concerns seriously, find another provider who will listen to you.

Understanding Your Body: Take the time to explore and learn about your body and what feels good for you. Knowing what feels right and what doesn't can help you communicate with your partner(s) during sexual activity.

Prioritizing Consent: Consent is crucial in any sexual encounter. It's important for women to feel in control of their bodies and to be able to give and receive enthusiastic consent.

Seeking Support: Having a supportive network of friends or professionals who understand and care about your sexual health can be invaluable. Don't hesitate to reach out for help to friends, family, or a therapist if you need support or guidance.

In conclusion, sexual health and safety are important aspects of our overall health and well-being. It's essential to prioritize our sexual health by regularly getting tested for

STIs, using contraceptives, practicing safe sex, seeking medical attention when necessary, and advocating for ourselves. By taking control of our sexual health and empowering ourselves, we can enjoy fulfilling and safe sexual experiences throughout our lives.

Chapter VIII.

Lifelong Sexual Fulfillment and Connection

Strategies for Maintaining Sexual Interest over Time

Maintaining a spark of sexual interest in a long-term relationship is essential for lifelong fulfillment and connection.

Here are some strategies for keeping the flame alive:

Prioritize Self-Exploration: Continue to explore your own desires and fantasies over time, and be willing to communicate them with your partner(s).

Cheryl Bach

Communication is Key: Open communication with your partner(s) about your sexual needs and experiences can build trust, intimacy, and understanding.

Mix it Up: Trying new activities and exploring different forms of sexual pleasure can break up monotony and add excitement to your sexual encounters.

Make Time for Sex: With busy schedules and obligations, it can be easy to let sex fall to the wayside. Schedule regular intimate time with your partner(s) to prioritize sexual connection and fulfillment.

The Importance of Intimacy and Connection in Sexual Relationships

Sexual connection is more than just physical pleasure – it's about creating a sense of intimacy and connection with your partner(s).

Here are some ways to foster that deeper connection:

Emotional Connection: Building an emotional connection with your partner(s) can create feelings of trust, security, and vulnerability. Take time to talk about your hopes and fears and share non-sexual activities together.

Sensory Experiences: Sensory experiences such as touching, tasting, and smelling can create a deeper sense of intimacy and bonding. Experiment with different kinds of touch, taste new foods, and use fragrance to create a sensual environment.

Non-Sexual Touch: Hugging, holding hands, and cuddling can be powerful ways of increasing intimacy and connection with your partner(s) and promote feelings of closeness and comfort.

Focusing on the Present Moment: During sexual encounters, focus on being present in the moment and enjoying the experience. Savor every touch, sensation, and emotion you feel.

Mutual Pleasure: Remember that sex should be a mutually pleasurable experience for both partners. Focus on exploring each other's bodies and finding what feels good.

Tips for Exploring New Fantasies and Desires over Time

Exploring new fantasies and desires can add excitement and novelty to your sexual experiences.

Here are some tips for doing so:

Start Small: Don't try to jump into anything too intense or out of your comfort zone right away. Start small and work your way up gradually.

Communicate Clearly: It's crucial to communicate openly and clearly with your partner(s) about your desires and boundaries. This can help prevent misunderstandings and ensure that both parties are comfortable with the activities.

Take Your Time: Exploring new fantasies or desires can be a process that takes time to explore. Be patient and don't rush into anything that doesn't feel right.

Do Your Research: If you are curious about a particular sexual activity, take time to research it before trying it. Learn about safety protocols and potential risks.

Try New Things Together: Explore new fantasies or desires with your partner(s). Trying new things together can promote feelings of bonding and connection.

Embracing Sexuality as a Vital Part of Overall Well-Being

Sexuality is not something to be ashamed of or ignored – it is an essential component of our overall well-being.

Here are some ways to embrace your sexuality:

Prioritize Sexual Health: Practice safe sex and get regular STI testing to ensure your sexual health.

Self-Love: Engage in self-love practices such as masturbation or connecting with your own body. This can help you better understand your desires and preferences.

Embrace Your Body: Our bodies change over time, but it's essential to embrace them and appreciate them for what they are. Developing a positive body image can foster a greater sense of sexual confidence.

Seek Support: If you are struggling with issues related to sexual desire, arousal, or function, seek out support from a healthcare professional or therapist who specializes in sexual health.

Remove Shame: Release any sense of shame or stigma you may feel about your sexuality. Understand that having positive sexual experiences is absolutely natural and can bring tremendous joy to your life.

In conclusion, lifelong sexual fulfillment and connection requires ongoing efforts in communication, intimacy, and exploration. Women can enjoy sexual fulfillment throughout their lives by being open to exploring new fantasies and desires, prioritizing emotional connection and physical touch, and seeing sexuality as an essential component of overall well-being. By following these tips and embracing their sexuality, women can experience deeper connections, greater pleasure, and a fulfilling sex life for the long-term.

Chapter IX.

Conclusion

Throughout this guide, we have explored various strategies and techniques for achieving multi-orgasmic sex, mastering pleasure, and embracing sexual empowerment. However, at the core of it all is the concept of prioritizing your own sexual well-being and happiness.

As women, we often receive messages from society that our sexuality should be repressed or stigmatized. We may feel guilty or ashamed for exploring our desires, or we may prioritize the needs and desires of others before our own. However, when it comes to sexuality, it's important to remember that you are the expert on your own body and what feels good for you.

By prioritizing your own needs and desires when it comes to sex, you can experience deeper connections, greater pleasure, and a more fulfilling sex life.

Here are some ways to do that:

Communicate Your Needs: It's crucial to be open and honest with your partner(s) about what feels good for you and what you need in order to experience pleasure. Don't be afraid to speak up and ask for what you want - your partner(s) will likely appreciate the guidance and will be happy to accommodate your needs.

Prioritize Self-Exploration: Take the time to explore your own body and learn what feels pleasurable for you. This can include solo exploration through masturbation or self-love practices, as well as experimenting with different forms of touch and stimulation during partnered sex.

Prioritize Your Own Pleasure: While it's important to consider your partner(s) needs and desires, don't neglect your own pleasure in the process. Take charge of your own sexual well-being and prioritize your own pleasure as a fundamental aspect of the sexual experience.

Embrace Your Desires: Don't be afraid to embrace your sexual desires, no matter how unconventional they may seem. Whether it's exploring kink and BDSM, experimenting with new forms of pleasure, or simply speaking up about what you want during sex, embracing your desires can lead to a more fulfilling and satisfying sex life.

Prioritize Sexual Health: It's important to prioritize your sexual health in order to fully enjoy your sexuality. This includes practicing safe sex, getting regular STI testing, and seeking support from healthcare professionals or therapists if struggling with sexual function or desire.

By prioritizing your own sexual well-being and happiness, you can achieve a more fulfilling and joyful sex life. Taking charge of your own desires and communicating your needs to your partner(s) can lead to deeper connections and greater pleasure. Embracing your sexuality as a natural and essential part of your overall well-being can help you achieve greater sexual fulfillment and lifelong intimate connection.

In conclusion, mastering multi-orgasmic sex is not just about physical techniques and strategies, but also about prioritizing your own sexual empowerment. By embracing your desires, communicating your needs, and taking charge of your own pleasure, you can achieve lifelong sexual fulfillment and intimate connection. I encourage women to experiment, explore, and prioritize their own sexual well-being and happiness above all else. Remember that your sexuality is a natural and fundamental aspect of who you are, and there is no shame in seeking pleasure and intimacy with yourself and others. Embrace your desires, master your pleasure, and enjoy the journey towards a more fulfilling and joyful sex life. Thank you for reading!

Cheryl Bach

www.ingramcontent.com/pod-product-compliance
Lightning Source LLC
Chambersburg PA
CBHW071551260726
48653CB00007BA/2790